SWEDISH MASSAGE

A Comprehensive Guide To Swedish Massage Techniques For Mental And Emotional Well-Being

NUEL NENJI

Contents

Introductory

Long, gliding strokes, kneading, and friction techniques are utilized in Swedish massage, a popular form of massage therapy that targets the lighter layers of muscle. Its intended benefits include circulation enhancement, muscle tension relief, and relaxation promotion.

Swing massage is distinguished by the following qualities:

• Long, arching strokes are utilized during effleurage to improve blood circulation and induce relaxation throughout the body.

- A form of muscle release and flexibility enhancement known as petrissage consists of kneading and compressing the muscles.

- In order to promote relaxation and dismantle adhesions, the therapist employs friction and pressure along the muscle's longitudinal axis.

- Tapotement is a form of stimulating the musculature and invigorating the body through the use of rhythmic tapping or percussive movements, such as hacking or cupping.

- Anxiety-relieving vibration or moderate shaking may be generated through the therapist's use of back-and-forth hand movements.

The delicate and calming characteristics of Swedish massage render it well-suited for individuals seeking relaxation rather than vigorous muscle engagement, as well as for those who are new to yoga.

Typically, the client rests on a massage table while the therapist applies oil or lotion to the skin to alleviate friction during sessions. This technique is prevalent in spa environments.

As a means of tailoring the session to your specific requirements, it is vital that you inform your massage therapist of your preferences and any particularized areas of concern or discomfort.

CHAPTER ONE
Positive Aspects Of Swedish Massage

Physical and mental health advantages are associated with Swedish massage. The following are some of the primary benefits:

• Comfort: Facilitating relaxation is the principal objective of Swedish massage. Stress and anxiety are alleviated through the calming effects of the soothing movements and delicate, flowing strokes.

• Blood circulation is enhanced throughout the body as a result of the lengthy, gliding strokes utilized in Swedish massage. Consequently, there is a potential for enhanced tissue oxygenation, improved nutrient transportation, and heightened muscle waste elimination efficiency.

• Muscle tension can be alleviated and pain reduced through the use of kneading and friction techniques in Swedish massage. Back pain, neck pain, and migraines are typical conditions that are frequently treated with it.

• Swedish massage has the potential to enhance flexibility and joint mobility through the promotion of relaxation and the targeting of muscle spasms. Individuals who have restricted range of motion or muscular tension can benefit significantly from this.

• Endorphins, the body's endogenous feel-good compounds, are released during massage therapy, which has been shown to improve mood. Enhanced mood and a heightened sense of well-being may result from this.

• Swedish massage has gained recognition for its acknowledged capacity to alleviate tension. It promotes mental health by simultaneously inducing relaxation and decreasing levels of the stress hormone cortisol.

• A Swedish massage has been reported to help numerous individuals achieve a higher quality of sleep. A deeper night's slumber may be facilitated by the relaxation that the massage induces.

• Swedish massage has the potential to enhance the body's method of eliminating waste products and pollutants through the promotion of lymphatic drainage and improved circulation.

• Regular Swedish massage, among other types of massage, may support the immune system by reducing tension and fostering general health, according to a number of studies.

It is crucial to acknowledge that reactions to massage can differ among individuals, and the aforementioned advantages might not be universally perceived.

Further, individuals with pre-existing health conditions or concerns should strongly consider seeking guidance from a healthcare professional prior to engaging in massage therapy.

Elements Constituting Swedish Massage

In order to facilitate a therapeutic and soothing experience, Swedish massage practitioners adhere to a number of foundational principles and techniques. Swedish massage is founded upon the following tenets:

- Effleurage, a Swedish massage technique of fundamental importance, comprises extensive, gliding strokes that are performed over the entirety of the body. Hands, fingertips, or forearms are commonly utilized to execute these motions.

In addition to promoting muscle warming and relaxation, effleurage facilitates the application of oil or ointment.

• Petrissage, which consists of pushing and compressing of tissues and muscles, is a form of kneading. Facilitating flexibility, enhancing circulation, and alleviating tension are all benefits of this method. Frequently, this entails the activation and contraction of the interdigital muscles.

• Pressure and rubbing motions along the muscle fibers' longitudinal axes constitute friction. By disintegrating connective tissue and muscle adhesions (knots), this method increases blood flow and flexibility in the muscles.

• Consisting of rhythmic striking, chopping, or pounding motions, tapotement is also known as rhythmic percussion. Muscle stimulation, overall body revitalization, and enhanced circulation are all potential outcomes of this method. Cupping, slicing, and tapping with the periphery of the hand are all typical tapotement activities.

• Vibration: The therapist practices vibration by producing a gentle shaking or vibrating motion with a back-and-forth movement of the hands or fingers. This method is frequently employed on particular regions and has the potential to alleviate muscular tension.

• Some Swedish massage therapists integrate range of motion exercises and light stretching into their therapeutic sessions. Flexibility and joint mobility are the objectives of these exercises.

• A continuous and rhythmic progression of movements

distinguishes Swedish massage. This seamless and pleasurable experience is facilitated by this flow, which contributes to the client's overall relaxation.

• Communication with and Comfort of the Client: Throughout the session, the therapist attends to the client's comfort.

To ensure that the pressure, techniques, and focal areas align with the client's preferences and requirements, an environment that promotes open communication is fostered.

• Oil or Lotion Application: Massage therapists frequently apply oil or lotion to the skin in order to reduce friction and improve the fluidity of strokes. Additionally, this facilitates the unimpeded movement of the therapist's palms across the client's physique.

• One client's particular requirements and inclinations may be accommodated through the adaptation of Swedish massage. Based on the client's objectives and health concerns, therapists may modify pressure, concentrate on specific areas of tension, and personalize the session.

Swedish massage is predicated on these tenets, which collectively promote physical and mental health while fostering a soothing and therapeutic environment.

CHAPTER TWO
A Variety Of Techniques And Strokes

Swedish massage optimizes circulation, induces relaxation, and alleviates tension through the application of a diverse array of strokes and techniques. The Swedish massage employs the following principal strokes and techniques:

• Long, gliding motions that encompass a substantial portion of the body constitute effleurage. Applying consistent pressure in the direction of blood flow toward the heart, the therapist utilizes their hands, palms, or forearms.

Beginning and concluding a massage session frequently involve effleurage.

• Petrissage consists of providing pressure to the muscles while rolling, kneading, and compressing them.

Muscle tissue is grasped and lifted by the therapist using their hands, fingertips, or thumbs. This method aids in the improvement of circulation, flexibility, and the relief of muscle tension.

• Utilizing circular or cross-fiber motions in conjunction with intense pressure constitute friction. Working on deeper layers of muscle and connective tissue, the therapist releases tension and dismantles adhesions by applying firm pressure to particular points.

• Consisting of rhythmic tapping, chopping, or hammering motions, tapotement is a form of percussion or rhythmic tapping.

Tipping with the fingertips, hacking (by utilizing the surfaces of the hands), and cupping (by forming a cup-like shape with the hand) are some variations. Body energizing, muscle-stimulating, and circulation-enhancing effects of tapotement.

• Vibration: The therapist practices vibration by producing a gentle shaking or vibrating motion with a back-and-forth movement of the hands or fingers. Relaxing tense muscles and enhancing circulation, this method is frequently administered to specific areas.

• Some Swedish massage therapists integrate range of motion exercises and light stretching into their therapeutic sessions. Flexibility, joint mobility, and general relaxation are the objectives of these exercises.

• Cross-fiber friction occurs when pressure is applied perpendicular to the direction of muscle fibers, as opposed to the typical friction experienced during normal movement. This may facilitate the disintegration of scar tissue, the liberation of adhesions, and the unification of muscles.

• Joint mobilization and stretching is a therapeutic technique employed by therapists to enhance the flexibility and range of motion of the joints through the use of mild movements.

• Utilizing the palms, hands, or fingers, consistent pressure is applied to a designated region during compression. Muscle tension can be alleviated and circulation can be enhanced.

• In order to alleviate pain and untangle muscle knots, trigger point therapy consists of the application of concentrated pressure to particular trigger points (localized areas of muscle tension).

With the client's requirements, preferences, and particularized areas of tension or discomfort in mind, therapists frequently integrate these strokes and techniques in a personalized fashion.

For a massage session to be both comfortable and effective, clients must be forthcoming with their massage therapist regarding any concerns or preferences they may have.

For Massage Therapists, Anatomy And Physiology

In order to guarantee secure and advantageous massage sessions for their clients, massage therapists must possess a comprehensive knowledge of anatomy and physiology. Anatomy and physiology fundamentals that are pertinent to massage therapy are summarized below:

1. System Muscular:

• Muscle anatomy knowledge, encompassing the origins, insertions, and functions of muscles.

• Familiarity with the functions of various muscle groups.

• Possess knowledge regarding prevalent muscle imbalances and patterns of tension.

2. Skeletal Body System:

• Knowledge of the anatomical arrangement and nomenclature of the bones comprising the body.

• Gaining insight into the structure and function of joints.

• Acknowledgement of prevalent collaborative concerns and circumstances.

3. System Nervous:

• Recognizing the composition and operation of the nervous system, encompassing both the peripheral and central nervous systems (including the brain and spinal cord).

• Physical and sensory pathway knowledge.

• Comprehension of the influence of the autonomic nervous system on stress reactions.

4. System of Circulation:

• Comprehending the heart, blood vessels, and blood as components of the cardiovascular system.

• A comprehension of the function of blood circulation in transporting nutrients and oxygen!

• The acknowledgment of prevalent cardiovascular ailments and factors to be taken into account when performing massage manipulations.

5. System Lymphatic:

• Comprehending the function of the lymphatic system within the context of the immune system.

• A comprehensive understanding of lymphatic drainage techniques to facilitate waste product removal.

6. System of Reciprocity:

• Knowledge of the structure and operation of the respiratory system, encompassing the lungs and bronchi.

- Knowledge of the significance of respiration in promoting relaxation and alleviating tension.

7. Skin: The Integumentary System

- Possessing knowledge of the functions of the skin's layers.

- Pronounced skin conditions and pertinent factors to be taken into account when performing massage techniques.

8. Systemic Endocrine:

- One must be cognizant of the function of the endocrine glands in producing hormones.

- I am aware of the potential effects that massage may have on hormone levels and the physiological effects that stress hormones have on the body.

9. System of Digestance:

- Extensive knowledge of the functions of the digestive organs.

- I am aware of any digestive issues that could potentially affect my massage sessions.

10. Calibration of Anatomy:

- Acquiring the ability to utilize palpation to evaluate joint mobility, muscle tension, and various other conditions affecting soft tissues.

- Recognizing the criticality of conducting effective client communication in order to pinpoint areas of concern or unease.

Additionally, in order to customize their approach for each client, massage therapists may investigate particular conditions, contraindications, and special populations. Therapists can refine their abilities and remain abreast of developments in the field by pursuing continuing education in anatomy and physiology. Furthermore, an extensive knowledge base in these areas enhances the professionalism and efficacy of massage therapy as a whole.

CHAPTER THREE
Establishment Of The Massage Environment

It is vital to establish the proper atmosphere prior to administering a massage in order to provide the client and massage therapist with a serene, professional, and comfortable setting.

Consider the following crucial steps:

1. Establishing the Massage Room:

• Inoculate, organize, and ventilate the massage chamber.

• Do so in order to achieve a comfortable temperature in the room. If a heating cloth is required for the massage table, consider employing one.

• Establish a tranquil ambiance by employing gentle, ambient lighting.

• To promote relaxation, dimly dimly select soothing music or natural noises.

2. Choose Sufficient Equipment:

• Towels, blankets, and sheets that are spotless and comfortable should be selectcd.

• Irrespective of the client's height, guarantee that the massage table is stable and appropriately adjusted.

• In order to ensure the client's comfort, ensure that an assortment of cushions and bolsters are accessible.

3.(Optional) Utilize Aromatherapy:

• One potential strategy to incorporate soothing fragrances into the space is by utilizing aromatherapy diffusers or essential oils.

• Ensure the client does not have any known allergies or sensitivities to particular fragrances by consulting them beforehand.

4. Implementing Effective Communication:

• Cordially and expertly greet the client.

• Inquire about the client's medical background, personal inclinations, and any particularized areas of apprehension.

• Assure the client is well-informed and at ease as you describe the massage procedure.

5. Ensure Privacy by:

• Inoculate the client in a tranquil and private area where they can undress and change.

• Isolate the client's personal possessions in a secure location.

6. Providing options for robes or drapes:

• The client may choose to wear a garment or another covering prior to and following the massage, if desired.

• Ensure the client feels secure and discreet while effectively conveying the draping protocol.

7. Encourage rituals prior to the massage:

• Prefer the client's comfort by advising them to utilize the restroom prior to the massage.

• Preach hydration by presenting a glass of water.

8. Establish an Ambiance of Relaxation:

• To reduce disruptions and external commotion.

• Establish a serene ambiance by incorporating soft, comfortable furnishings and décor.

9. Assess Comfort Levels:

• Investigate with the client any additional factors that may be influencing their wellbeing, such as the room temperature and pressure.

• In accordance with the client's preferences, modify any components, including the volume of the music or the illumination.

10. Establish Boundaries Proficiently:

• Communicate expectations and boundaries in a professional manner.

- If the client has any concerns or requires adjustments during the massage, emphasize the value of open communication.

Spa clinicians can cultivate an atmosphere that promotes relaxation and therapeutic advantages by attending to these particulars, thereby assisting clients in feeling comfortable.

Personalized and amicable massage experiences are the result of the therapist's awareness and sensitivity to the preferences of each individual client.

Essential Elements Of Swedish Massage

In this well-known massage technique, Swedish massage strokes serve as the basis. In Swedish massage, the following are the foundational strokes:

1. Long glider strokes constitute effleurage:

• To stretch the client's skin, apply oil or lotion, and warm up the musculature are the intended results.

• Long, fluid motions in the direction of blood flow toward the heart, executed with the hands, palms, or forearms.

2. Kneading: Petrissage

• To enhance circulation, facilitate flexibility, and alleviate muscle tension are the intended effects.

• To elevate and compress muscle tissue, the technique involves performing rolling, squeezing, and kneading movements with the hands, fingers, or thumbs.

3. In friction:

• To increase circulation, disentangle adhesions, and alleviate tension in deeper muscle layers.

• Methodology: Employ firm pressure to execute circular or cross-fiber motions utilizing the fingertips, thumbs, or palms.

4. Constriction or Percussion (Tapotement):

• The objective is to improve circulation, stimulate muscles, and invigorate the body.

Methods include:

• Cupping: rhythmically tapping the body while forming a cup-like shape with the palm.

• Hacking: Executing rhythmic chopping motions with the sides of the forearms.

• Tapping: A rhythmic action involving the application of fingertips to the body.

5. The vibration

• Goal: To facilitate comprehensive relaxation and alleviate tension in the muscles.

• Method: Generate a mild vibration or shaking sensation by employing a back-and-forth motion of the hands or fingertips.

Swedish massage consists of a sequence of these fundamental strokes that are frequently combined and utilized in a comprehensive manner.

Furthermore, in accordance with the client's inclinations and requirements, clinicians may modify the pressure and methodologies. An overall sense of well-being and relaxation is induced by the cadence and flow of the strokes.

It is noteworthy that although the aforementioned strokes form the basis of Swedish massage, proficient therapists may integrate modifications and adaptations in accordance with the specific needs of each client. A positive experience and the customization of the massage to the client's comfort require that the therapist and client maintain clear and concise communication.

CHAPTER FOUR
Orders And Routines Of Massage

To ensure a thorough and effective massage, massage therapists frequently employ predetermined sequences and routines throughout sessions.

The variety of massage performed, the client's requirements, and the therapist's level of training may influence these sequences. A Swedish massage sequence, a widely employed and adaptable technique, can be succinctly described as follows.

1. Consultation and Preface:

Cordially welcome the client.

• In order to address the client's specific concerns, preferences, and health history, it is imperative to conduct a concise consultation.

• Assist with inquiries and describe the massage procedure.

2. In the beginning, Effleurage:

• Introduce oil or lotion onto the skin while performing effleurage strokes to warm up the muscles.

• Move the entire body with extended, gliding strokes.

3. Aspects of Petrissage:

• Knead and compress the muscles while transitioning to petrissage techniques.

• Emphasize areas of tension and main muscle groups.

4. Damaged by friction:

• To target deeper muscle layers and effectively eliminate adhesions, integrate friction strokes.

• Implement firm pressure while performing circular or cross-fiber movements.

5. Vibration and Acupointment:

• To generate muscle stimulation, incorporate tapotement techniques including hacking, tapping, and cupping.

• One way to induce relaxation is by incorporating vibration movements.

6. Work on Particular Muscles:

• Objective techniques are designed to target particular muscles or areas of tension.

• Petrissage, friction, or kneading should be utilized further if necessary.

7. Range of motion and stretching:

• Strengthen flexibility by incorporating range-of-motion exercises and light stretching.

• Consider the comfort and level of flexibility of the client.

8. Supplementary Joint Mobilization:

• For the purpose of augmenting joint mobility, incorporate joint mobilization techniques.

• Employ deliberate and subdued motions.

9. Effervescence as a final:

• Revert to effleurage strokes gradually thereafter.

• In order to conclude the massage in a tranquil and pleasing manner.

10. Suggestions and Feedback Following the Massage:

• Inquire with the client regarding their experience-related feedback.

• Provide recommendations for post-massage care, including stretching exercises and hydration.

Notably, massage therapists frequently modify their techniques in accordance with the specific requirements and preferences of each client. Thus, this sequence should be regarded as a broad approximation. In addition to aromatherapy, deep tissue work, and hot stone massage, some therapists may integrate specialized techniques and additional modalities into their practices.

The therapist can achieve the intended therapeutic outcomes and better suit the client's comfort level by maintaining open lines of communication with the client throughout the session.

Avoidance And Precautionary Measures

In order to safeguard their clients' health and safety, massage therapists must give due regard to contraindications and precautionary measures.

Precautions involve modifying the massage approach to address particular concerns, whereas contraindications are conditions or circumstances in which massage is not advised.

In order to ascertain any contraindications or precautions prior to commencing a massage session, it is imperative that massage therapists conduct a comprehensive client consultation. Examples of this are typical:

Indications against use:

1. Conditions of Infectious Skin:

- Skin infections, blemishes, or contagious conditions are considered contraindications.

- One potential consequence of massage is the exacerbation or transmission of the infection.

2. Acute Illness or Fever:

- Flu, fever, or other acute illnesses are contraindications.

- Owing to the tension caused by illness, massage may place additional strain on a body that is already strained.

3. Cardiovascular conditions that are severe:

- Uncontrolled hypertension, a recent myocardial infarction, or severe myocardial conditions are contraindications.

- Certain cardiovascular conditions may render individuals more susceptible to the effects of massage on blood pressure.

4. Venous deep vein thrombosis (DVT):

• Active DVT or a previous predisposition to blood clotting are contraindications.

• One potential reason for the risk of complications is that massage may disturb a thrombus.

5. Critical respiratory illnesses include:

• Asthma, pneumonia, or severe respiratory distress constitute contraindications.

• Breathing difficulties may be further aggravated by the strain placed on the respiratory system during a massage.

6. Trauma or Severe Pain:

• Recent fractures, injuries, or acute pain are contraindications.

• Therapy may exacerbate the condition or induce additional damage.

7. Preferred Pharmaceuticals:

• Contraindications include certain analgesics, blood-thinning drugs, or blood pressure-regulating medications.

• These medications have the potential to elevate the likelihood of experiencing adverse reactions, bruising, or hemorrhaging.

8. Particular Skin Disorders:

• Open incisions, burns, or extensive skin injuries are considered contraindications.

• Massage could potentially exacerbate or cause irritation to the condition.

Risks to Consider:

1. The Obstructure:

• Strict caution is recommended and specific positions should be avoided throughout the initial trimester.

- Why: To guarantee the comfort and security of both the developing embryo and the mother.

2. Disorders of Chronic Health:

- Care should be taken when performing massage techniques on individuals with conditions such as cancer, diabetes, or arthritis, as they may necessitate modifications.

- Justification: In order to tailor the massage to the particular requirements and constraints of the client.

3.   Contemporary   Surgical Procedures:

• Owing to recent surgical procedures, massage should be modified or avoided.

• For the purpose of averting distress or complications during the healing process.

4. Phosphates of the bone:

• Avoid vigorous joint movements and apply gentle pressure as a precaution.

• As a precaution against possible fractures of fragile bones.

5. Senior Customers:

- Regarding potential frailty, exercise caution and employ gentle techniques.

- Motive: To ensure that elderly individuals have a secure and pleasant experience.

To ensure a safe and beneficial massage experience, clinicians ought to consult healthcare professionals when uncertain and collaborate with clients.

CHAPTER FIVE
Particular Populations Receiving Massage

Special populations—individuals with particular health conditions or life circumstances—may have massage therapy modified to accommodate their particular requirements and circumstances. Massage techniques tailored to special populations include the following:

1. Massage Prenatal:

- Attention: Modified to accommodate expectant women.

• Take into account the following: adopt a lateral position, prevent pressure on specific areas, and attend to frequent pregnancy discomforts.

• Advantages: Anti-estrus, circulation, and relaxation enhancements throughout the course of pregnancy.

2. Massage for the elderly:

• To be taken into account are age-related conditions such as osteoporosis or arthritis, the need for gentle pressure, and the ability to accommodate physical limitations.

- Aging-related benefits include increased circulation, improved joint mobility, and relaxation.

3. Massage for Pediatrics:

- Opinions: Reduced session durations, child-friendly surroundings, and the implementation of mild techniques.

- Children coping with medical conditions or tension will experience reduced anxiety, enhanced sleep, and relaxation.

4. Patients with Cancer:

• Supporting patients who are enduring cancer treatment is the primary objective.

• Care should be taken to modify pressure in accordance with treatment-related adverse effects, prevent contact with affected areas, and secure appropriate medical approval.

• Treatment-related symptoms are alleviated, anxiety is reduced, and sleep quality is enhanced.

5. Body Massage for Hospice and Palliative Care:

• Owing to the fact that it provides solace to those afflicted with life-limiting ailments.

• Factors to Consider: Supporting the individual emotionally, employing a gentle contact, and accommodating their comfort level.

6. Members of the gymnasium:

• The primary audience consists of athletics enthusiasts.

• Considerations: recuperation support, targeting particular muscle groups, and stretching integration.

• Improved athletic performance, decreased muscle fatigue, and enhanced flexibility are some of the benefits.

7. Chronically Painful Clients:

• Owing to persistent discomfort conditions, this is the aim.

• One should take into account the level of discomfort and concentrate on specific areas of tension when adjusting pressure and techniques.

• Relaxation, enhanced range of motion, and a diminished perception of discomfort are notable advantages.

8. Sufferers of Depression and Anxiety:

• Enhancing mental health and well-being is the primary objective.

• It is advisable to establish a serene ambiance, integrate relaxation strategies, and employ delicate brushstrokes.

• Advantages: tranquility, reduced symptoms of anxiety and depression, and enhanced mood.

9. Disorders of the nervous system (such as Parkinson's and multiple sclerosis):

- Owing to the fact that it targets particular symptoms linked to neurological disorders.

- Modifying methodologies to accommodate unique mobility capacities and individual requirements.

- Additional advantages include enhanced relaxation, improved circulation, and decreased muscle stiffness.

10. Individuals with a history of trauma:

- Stakeholders with trauma are offered a secure and encouraging environment.

• Considerations: employing gentle and non-invasive techniques, ensuring adequate assent is obtained, and communicating clearly.

• Safety, enhanced body awareness, and decreased anxiety are some of the benefits.

It is imperative that the massage therapist and client maintain unambiguous communication in all circumstances. A secure and effective session for special populations can be achieved through the following: acquiring a comprehensive health history, recognizing their unique needs and concerns, and adjusting the massage techniques accordingly. Furthermore, specific medical conditions may require the involvement of other healthcare professionals in partnership.

Massage Therapists' Exercise In Self-Care

The maintenance of one's physical, mental, and emotional well-being is of the utmost importance for massage therapists. Therapists must also prioritize their own health, despite the fact that their profession entails offering assistance and care to others.

Massage therapists may integrate the following self-care practices into their daily routines:

1. Consistent Physical Upkeep:

• One way to support muscle strain and preserve flexibility is to incorporate stretching exercises into your routine on a regular basis.

• To ensure appropriate body mechanics during massages, strengthen the core muscles through strength training.

• To alleviate any tension or distress, establish a routine for yourself to receive massages.

2. Mechanics of the Body Proper:

• To mitigate self-inflicted strain on the body, ensure that you maintain proper posture while receiving massages.

• Engaging in regular body mechanics training is a worthwhile investment of time in order to enhance one's physical prowess and acquire knowledge of strategies to reduce muscular strain.

3. Recuperation Rest:

• Irrespective of energy levels and general well-being, it is imperative that you obtain sufficient restorative slumber.

• To facilitate my recovery from the physical demands of massage therapy, it is recommended that I include leisure days in my schedule.

4. Supplements and Hydration:

• To maintain proper hydration, which is vital for overall health, consume sufficient water throughout the day.

• To furnish your body with the essential nutrients required for energy production and recuperation, it is imperative to consume a balanced diet.

5. Psychological Health:

• Conducting routine self-reflection and emotional well-being check-ins should be a priority for you.

• If necessary, contemplate obtaining therapeutic support from a counselor or therapist.

6. Organization of Time:

• Originate Limitations: To prevent exhaustion, establish distinct limitations between one's professional and personal spheres.

• In order to guarantee sufficient time for work, self-care, and personal activities, it is essential to effectively manage your schedule.

7. Practicing the Mind-Body:

• One effective approach to alleviating tension and enhancing mental health is to integrate mindfulness or meditation techniques into one's routine.

• One can enhance flexibility, balance, and relaxation by participating in mind-body disciplines such as yoga or Tai Chi.

8. Recreation and Hobbies:

• Owing to their capacity to elicit pleasure and facilitate creative expression, engage in pastimes or pursuits that are creative in nature.

• To decompress and have fun, schedule time for enjoyable recreational activities.

9. Prolonged Education:

• Continuous learning and professional development are essential for individuals to augment their expertise and understanding.

• To foster support and facilitate the exchange of knowledge, establish connections with other massage therapists or healthcare professionals.

10. Sufficient Intervals for Work:

• Scheduled Breaks: It is imperative that you incorporate periodic rest and recharging breaks into your workday.

• One way to prevent overwork of particular muscle groups is to incorporate a variety of massage techniques into each session.

In addition to providing personal benefits, prioritizing self-care enhances the therapist's ability to deliver high-quality care to their clients. To ensure the longevity and satisfaction of their profession, massage therapists must acknowledge and attend to their personal requirements.

Summary

A variety of physical, mental, and emotional benefits are provided by massage therapists and clients, constituting an all-encompassing approach to health and well-being. The discipline of massage therapists emphasizes the significance of self-care in addition to the traditional Swedish massage techniques that promote relaxation, tension reduction, and overall health support.

This diversity is reflected in the specialized modalities designed for specific populations and the fundamental techniques of Swedish massage.

In addition to improving circulation, facilitating flexibility, and alleviating specific conditions, massage therapy offers clients a means to alleviate tension. Massage is a versatile and commonly embraced form of complementary healthcare due to its adaptability, which permits customization according to individual requirements.

An instruction in diverse massage techniques, anatomy, and

physiology is fundamental to the profession of massage therapy. Complementing effective communication skills with the capacity to establish a nurturing and tranquil atmosphere guarantees that clients are at ease and derive optimal advantages from their therapeutic sessions.

Additionally, massage therapists must recognize the critical nature of self-care. A sustainable and satisfying career is enhanced by consistent physical hygiene, correct body mechanics, adequate rest, and emotional well-being. Massage therapists can ensure the perpetuation of their profession and the provision of high-quality services to their customers by placing self-care as a top priority.

Fundamentally, massage therapy is a field characterized by its constant improvement and incorporation of novel techniques and information. The continued importance of massage therapy in facilitating relaxation, mitigating pain, and bolstering general wellness persists as more people pursue holistic approaches to health and well-being.

THE END